Fibromyalgia

The complete guide to Fibromyalgia, and how to treat and overcome it!

Table of Contents

Introduction

Thank you for taking the time to pick up this book about Fibromyalgia. This book aims to serve as a guide to Fibromyalgia, educating you on the condition and helping you to better understand how it can be treated.

Being considered a chronic disease, there is no current cure for Fibromyalgia. However, there are many ways to improve the condition, and reduce symptoms.

Throughout the following chapters, you will learn about how Fibromyalgia is diagnosed, what the different symptoms are, how it is treated with Western medicine, and how you can treat it with some alternative therapies and dietary changes.

Once again, thanks for choosing this book, I hope you find it to be helpful!

Chapter 1: What is Fibromyalgia?

Fibromyalgia is a chronic disorder that causes widespread musculoskeletal pain, fatigue, sleeping problems, memory issues, and depression, among other issues. People with this condition also have areas of tenderness or tender points which ache when pressure is placed on them. Researchers believe that the brain of a person with fibromyalgia amplifies pain signals, resulting in constant and sometimes extreme pain in the muscles even when there is no apparent injury or cause.

Prevalence

Fibromyalgia affects more than 5 million Americans aged 18 years old and above. More than half of this number is women. However, men and younger people can also develop the disorder. Most fibromyalgia patients are diagnosed during their middle age.

Fibromyalgia vs. Chronic Fatigue Syndrome

Fibromyalgia and Chronic Fatigue Syndrome (CFS) are similar in many ways and share many similar symptoms such as pain and fatigue. In fact, it is common for an individual to have both conditions. Some medical experts believe that CFS and fibromyalgia are the same disorder, only expressed in somewhat different ways.

Both fibromyalgia and CFS can be debilitating and negatively impact day-to-day life. The characterizing symptom of CFS is extreme tiredness or fatigue that isn't caused by any underlying medical condition, and that doesn't go away with rest or sleep. CFS often starts with flu-like symptoms and later causes other disturbing signs. Aside from severe tiredness, a person with CFS experiences at least 4 of the following:

- Aches or pain in the joints without redness or swelling

- Muscle aches or pain

- Feeling exhausted even after a long sleep

- Having difficulty focusing and remembering things

- Unusual headaches (of a new pattern, strength, or type)

- Tender lymph nodes under the arms or in the neck

- Having an uncomfortable or "out-of-short" feeling after being physically active

- Sore throat

Unlike fibromyalgia, CFS patients do not have trigger or tender points.

Cure for Fibromyalgia

There is presently no cure for fibromyalgia, as researchers and doctors don't understand what exactly causes it. Treatment, which involves medication, therapy, self-care, and lifestyle changes, focuses on reducing symptoms and improving the patient's quality of life.

As it is a chronic condition, fibromyalgia lasts for a long period of time, most possibly a lifetime. But on a lighter note, this condition is not progressive and is never fatal. It may cause pain but will not damage the muscles, joints, or internal organs. Though it isn't currently curable, fibromyalgia improves over time with proper care, treatment, and management.

Chapter 2: Causes and Symptoms

Causes

The exact cause of fibromyalgia is not known. However, doctors and medical researchers believe a number of factors may be working together to trigger it. These risk factors include:

- **Genetics**: Fibromyalgia appears to run in families. People whose family has a history of the condition have a higher risk of developing it. Certain genetic mutations may be responsible for this. However, those genes have yet to be identified.

- **Infections/Diseases**: Certain illnesses may trigger or worsen the symptoms of fibromyalgia. Rheumatic diseases like rheumatoid arthritis and lupus may also increase risk.

- **Physical/Emotional trauma**: Being exposed to emotional or physical trauma can develop fibromyalgia. These include car accidents and repetitive injuries (injuries to the body resulting from doing the same action repeatedly).

- **Psychological stress**: Psychological stress can be the result of stressful events like experiencing major accidents, assaults, or time spent at war. It has been associated with hormonal disturbances which can contribute to the development of the condition. Like trauma, phycological stress can produce far-reaching effects to the body which can linger for months and even years. Fibromyalgia has been linked to PTSD or post-traumatic stress disorder.

- **Gender**: Statistics show that women are more susceptible to fibromyalgia. According to the National Institute of Arthritis and Musculoskeletal and Skin Diseases (NIAMS), women make up 80 to 90% of all fibromyalgia cases. The reasons behind this are not known.

A theory suggests that fibromyalgia can be caused by the receptors and nerves in the body becoming more sensitive to stimulus. This means they misinterpret or overreact to the pain signals, causing exaggerated or unnecessary pain. Another theory suggests that it may be due to the brain lowering the pain threshold. So what used to cause no pain causes extreme pain as time goes by. Others suggest that it may be caused by certain chemical imbalances in the brain.

Symptoms

In some cases, symptoms of fibromyalgia begin after a major psychological stress, physical trauma, surgery, or infection. In others, symptoms accumulate gradually with time, with not a single triggering event.

Pain and Tender/Trigger Points

Widespread joint and muscle pain is one of the classic symptoms of fibromyalgia. The pain is often described as a dull, deep, sharp, throbbing ache persisting for at least 3 months. Widespread means it occurs on both sides of the body, and below and above the waist. In other words, the ache is all over.

The pain is quite similar to bursitis, tendinitis, and osteoarthritis, but it is felt all over the body—in the tendons, muscles, and ligaments surrounding the joints. The pain may come and go, but in many cases, it is constant.

People with fibromyalgia also have areas of tenderness, called tender or trigger points. These are specific places on the body, usually around the joints, that hurt when being pressed with a finger. However, it isn't the joints that hurt, but the tissue around them. People without fibro will only feel pressure when you press these tender points. But for those with fibro, even light pressure on those points can cause severe pain.

Trigger points often include:

- tops of shoulders

- back of the head

- upper chest

- knees hips

- outer elbows

There are 18 known trigger points, and a person with fibro has at least 11. Doctors rarely use tender points to diagnose fibromyalgia, but they use them to narrow down the list of other possible diagnoses.

Fatigue

Another classic symptom of fibromyalgia is fatigue—that constant feeling of tiredness and exhaustion, even when they should be feeling well rested (such as after sleeping for a long period of time). Some people say it's like having the flu or it's as if you missed a lot of sleep or worked long hours.

If you have fibro, you may also feel too tired to work out or more exhausted after a normal exercise. Even the easiest tasks like ironing or folding clothes can become painful. Simple activities such as going on a simple errand, shopping, or cooking dinner can drain you and make you feel all wiped out.

Sleep problems

Pain often disrupts sleep. And when you are able to sleep, it is usually light and easily interrupted. Many people with fibromyalgia also suffer from other sleep disorders like sleep apnea and restless leg syndrome.

According to tests conducted in sleep laboratories, fibro patients are constantly disturbed by surges of brain activity which also occur when they are awake. These disturbances limit the time spent in deep sleep, resulting in a constant knocked-out feeling.

Mood Disorders

Having to deal with consistent pain and fatigue can lead to stress and mood problems. Patients may be anxious about how they will carry on with life, or worry about never feeling better. They may also tend to reduce social interactions and physical activities, resulting in self-isolation and depression.

Up to 50% of fibromyalgia patients have anxiety or depression, or both. It may be possible that these mood disorders, like pain, are part of the condition.

People diagnosed with depression and fibromyalgia also have difficulty focusing, remembering things, paying attention, and concentrating on mental tasks. This is referred to as "fibro fog."

Headaches

About 2 of 5 people with fibromyalgia suffer from tension headaches or migraines regularly. This can be triggered by pain in the upper back and neck, which is caused by the tightening of muscles in the area. Headaches can also be due to the tender points on the neck and back of the head.

Irritable Bowel Syndrome

Irritable bowel syndrome or IBS is a functional digestive disorder marked by altered bowel movements and abdominal stress. Up to two-thirds of fibro patients experience IBS symptoms such as stomach pain, bloating, nausea, and gas.

Many also have gastro-esophageal reflux disease (GERD) and acid reflux.

Morning Stiffness

People with fibromyalgia wake up with morning stiffness similar to what a person with rheumatoid arthritis feels. The stiffness occurs in the joints and muscles of the arms, legs, and back. For some people, it lasts only for a few minutes, but for most, it persists for more than 20 minutes each day. It sometimes lingers for hours, and possibly even all day. This makes it harder for fibro patients to start their day or get through it.

Paresthesia

Many fibromyalgia patients experience paresthesia, which is a burning, prickling, swelling, or tingling sensation usually felt in the arms, hands, legs, and feet. Its real cause is unclear but it is often a symptom of an underlying nerve damage or neurological disease. For someone with fibro, the burning or tingling sensation may be felt constantly, or just for a few minutes at random times. Though paresthesia is painless, it can be troublesome especially when it strikes in the morning along with morning stiffness.

Menstrual Cramps

Women are ten times more likely to develop fibromyalgia than men. And some of those affected women suffer more severe pain and symptoms once per month—that is, during their menstrual period. According to the National Fibromyalgia Association, women with fibro experience more painful menstrual cramps than normal. The pain sometimes fluctuates with their cycle, but the overall sensitivity and pain is heightened.

Problems Urinating

If you have fibromyalgia, you may feel constant urge to urinate, experience pain or lack of control when urinating, or have a leaky bladder. These symptoms may also be caused by a kidney and bladder infection or disease. Women with fibro tend to be more prone to these bladder control problems.

Restless Legs Syndrome

Restless legs syndrome, otherwise known as Willis-Ekbom Disease, is a condition that causes an irresistible urge to move your legs due to uncomfortable or unpleasant sensations in your lower legs and feet. The feeling is often described as crawling or tingling in nature and is most severe when you're at rest, either lying down or sitting. This can be especially bothersome at night as it can make it harder for you to sleep.

In addition, people with fibromyalgia may also have temporomandibular joint (TMJ) disorders and increased sensitivity to temperatures, bright lights, and loud noises. No imaging or lab test can detect this condition, so it is important to tell your doctor all your symptoms to get an accurate diagnosis.

Chapter 3: Diagnosis and Treatment

Diagnosis

Since the main symptoms of fibromyalgia, i.e., widespread pain and fatigue, aren't distinctive and can be symptoms of many other medical conditions, it is often misunderstood and misdiagnosed. You may have the condition but do not manifest all the symptoms, or you may have other medical problems that mimic the symptoms of fibro.

For these reasons and also due to the fact that the condition cannot be detected by lab tests, it often takes seeing several doctors before you can are diagnosed with fibromyalgia. The doctor may start the diagnosis based upon these two criteria:

- Widespread pain: Pain can be considered a symptom if it has lasted for at least 3 months with no identifiable cause. The pain must be felt in both left and right sides of your body, and below and above the waist.

- Presence of trigger/tender points: The doctor will press firmly on the 18 specific spots on your body to check how many of them are painful. You may feel pain in other places, but only those 18 spots can be used for diagnosis. You must have 11 or more tender points to be diagnosed with fibromyalgia.

The doctor may conduct some tests to rule out other medical conditions that may be triggering your symptoms, such as rheumatoid arthritis, multiple sclerosis, sleep apnea, and lupus. These tests can include blood tests which may involve:

- Total blood count

- Cyclic citrullinated peptide test

- Erythrocyte sedimentation rate

- Thyroid function test

- Rheumatoid factor

In addition, your doctor may ask if you've been having trouble sleeping or been feeling anxious and depressed. For a more precise diagnosis, prepare for your doctor's appointment by creating a list of the following:

- All your symptoms with detailed descriptions

- Information about your past medical problems

- Information about your family's medical history

- All medications and supplements you're taking, if any

- Any questions you may want to ask your doctor

Tell your doctor everything. Leaving out any information can make a big difference in your final diagnosis.

Treatment

Treating fibromyalgia generally includes medication and self-care. The emphasis is to minimize symptoms and improve general health and quality of life. No single treatment tackles all symptoms.

Treatment may also require a team of medical specialists with different expertise. This may include your physician or doctor, a rheumatologist, a physical therapist, and other healthcare providers.

A common treatment approach may include the following:

Medications and Supplements

Medications can provide relief from pain and improve mood and quality of sleep. Common medications for fibro include:

- Pain relievers: Three medications have been approved by the Food and Drug Administration (FDA) for the treatment of fibromyalgia. These are milnacipran (Savella), duloxetine (Cymbalta), and pregabalin (Lyrica). Over-the-counter painkillers such as acetaminophen (Tylenol), naproxen sodium (Aleve), and ibuprofen (Advil) may also be helpful. These drugs can help promote sleep, reduce inflammation, and minimize overall aches.

  For extreme cases, your doctor may prescribe tramadol (Ultram), to be used with caution so as to reduce risks of side effects and dependence. Narcotics are not recommended as these can aggravate pain over time and lead to addiction.

- Antidepressants: Your doctor may also advise low-dose antidepressants to help reduce aches, fatigue, anxiety and/or depression, and promote better sleep. Milnacipran (Savella) and duloxetine (Cymbalta) also fall under the antidepressant category. You may also be prescribed cyclobenzaprine (muscle relaxant), or amitriptyline to ease discomfort and lift your mood.

  Antidepressants can cause unpleasant side-effects such as nausea, loss of libido, and weight gain. Discuss possible repercussions with your doctor.

- Anticonvulsants: Drugs for treating epilepsy can be useful in lowering pain levels. FDA-approved pregabalin (Lyrica) is the first anti-seizure medicine for the treatment of fibromyalgia. Gabapentin (Neurontin) may also help in reducing symptoms. However, these drugs may come with some side-effects such as dry mouth, dizziness, swelling, and weight gain.

- Vitamin D: Fibro patients often have low vitamin D levels. In a 2013 study, people with fibromyalgia reported experiencing less fatigue and feeling physically better after taking vitamin D supplements regularly. Speak with your doctor about taking this supplement for proper implementation. Too much of the vitamin can become toxic.

Complementary Therapies

Along with medications, you can incorporate complementary therapies to relieve your symptoms. Alternative remedies help reduce pain, lower stress levels, and make you feel better overall. Discuss the following options with your doctor:

- Physical therapy

  PT techniques are intended to strengthen your muscles, improve your stamina, flexibility, and range of motion, and in turn reduce your pain. Your physical therapist can also teach you self-care techniques to help you manage pain and fatigue on your own.

- Occupational therapy

  An occupational therapy program can improve your functional abilities, confidence, and overall quality of life. Your therapist will help you make modifications to your work area or to the way you carry out certain tasks in order to minimize the stress brought upon your body.

- Massage therapy

  A good massage relaxes the muscles, reduces tension, eases anxiety and stress, and enhances your range of motion. If too much pressure is applied, you may experience temporary swelling, bruising, and pain, so make sure to hire the right massage therapist for your condition.

- Cognitive behavior therapy

  CBT aims to help patients identify and modify maladaptive beliefs and behaviors, develop techniques to manage negative thought patterns, increase self-efficacy for pain management, and improve overall physical function. It is also used to cope with anxiety, depression, and sleep problems.

- Aromatherapy

  The therapeutic benefits of essential oils can be extremely helpful in relieving pain, fatigue, and cognitive issues. The best oils for this purpose include lavender, peppermint, helichrysum (everlasting flowers), jasmine, roman chamomile, ginger, eucalyptus, juniper, rosemary, neroli, and marjoram.

- Myofascial release therapy

  MFR therapy stimulates stretch reflex, relaxes contracted muscles, and improves lymphatic and blood circulation to treat pain and muscle immobility, and restore motion. This is done by applying sustained pressure into the connective tissues (fascia) in the muscles.

- Biofeedback

  Through biofeedback, you get to monitor your bodily functions, such as heart rate and blood pressure through sensors, and learn how to control them to your advantage. This technique can help you relax and control tension headaches among other symptoms. One form of biofeedback that is helpful for fibro patients is electromyography, which reads your body for muscle shortening or spasms.

- Light aerobics

  Light aerobic exercises such as walking, running, biking, and swimming, are some of the best ways to tackle your fibro symptoms. These exercises are simple and don't require any special equipment. Aerobic exercises use the large muscle groups for a set period of time. This releases the tension in the muscles while strengthening them. A 2017 review found that aerobic exercises can improve pain and stiffness, muscle function, and quality of life.

- Water exercise

  Water-based therapy, or water aerobics, is an easy yet effective exercise for anyone suffering from chronic pain. It gets blood flow to your tendons and muscles to help alleviate pain and muscle tension. And since you're in the water, you aren't stressing your joints during the exercise. The buoyancy of the water also helps with movement. Note: You don't necessarily need to know how to swim to join a water aerobics class.

- Acupuncture

  This practice involves puncturing the skin with super fine needles to help improve blood flow, foster natural self-healing, restore chemical balance in the brain, and thereby treat chronic pain and a number of other health problems. The risks of this practice may include bruising, soreness, and minor bleeding. Make sure the acupuncturist you hire is a licensed professional.

- Acupressure

  If you don't like the idea of pricking your skin with needles, then you can try acupressure. This uses similar principles as acupuncture but instead of using needles, the practitioner uses their fingers, palm, elbows, or feet to apply pressure onto the acupoints on your body's meridians. Special devices may also be used in the practice.

- Relaxation techniques

  Relaxation techniques include mindfulness practice, slow breathing, and many forms of meditation. These practices stimulate the parasympathetic nervous system to help relieve your symptoms.

- Tai chi

  Tai chi is a Chinese martial art that fosters mind-body awareness, so it can help with both the psychological and physical symptoms of fibromyalgia. It involves deep meditation, controlled movements, and deep breathing. This practice can enhance your balance, muscle strength, and stamina. While it is not vigorous, you may develop sprains or sore muscles if you overdo it.

- Qigong

  Pronounced *chee-gong*, qigong is another ancient Chinese practice that has been shown to improve energy, ease pain, and lessen fatigue in several studies. This practice combines dance, movement, breathing techniques, and meditation.

- Yoga

  Research shows that people with fibromyalgia who joined yoga classes improved their mood and experienced less fatigue and overall pain. The practice improves muscle strength, and teaches a variety of relaxation techniques. The classes typically include gentle poses, breathing exercises, meditation, and group discussions. If you're joining a yoga class, be sure to tell the instructor that you have fibromyalgia so he or she can modify the poses as necessary for you.

Other Alternative Treatments

- Medicinal herbs and nutritional supplements

  Certain traditional herbs have been used for the treatment of fibromyalgia symptoms. These include grape seed extract, Siberian ginseng, valerian oil or root, and St. John's wort tincture. Supplements such as magnesium, melatonin, and SAMe have also been shown to aid the condition.

- Chiropractic or osteopathic manipulation

  These are nonsurgical treatment options for chronic pain. They are typically used for back pain but may also be beneficial for people with fibromyalgia. These procedures attempt to relieve pain by balancing muscle and tissue mechanics, and improving the range of motion of the joints.

- Medical marijuana

  One study discovered that people with fibromyalgia who took medical cannabis experienced reduced pain and stiffness, increased sleepiness, improved relaxation, mental abilities and sense of wellbeing. However, further research is needed to support the benefits and long-term effects of medicinal cannabis for the treatment of fibromyalgia.

In all cases, discuss with your doctor the possible upsides and downsides of each treatment approach before trying them.

Chapter 4: Coping Strategies

Self-care is crucial in the management of fibromyalgia. While there is no cure for this disorder, there are many strategies you can implement on a daily basis to cope with the symptoms and improve your condition. Consider the following.

De-stress

It is now known that stress can trigger symptoms of fibromyalgia. Allow yourself some time to unwind each day. Develop a plan to limit or avoid emotional stress and overexertion. This may include saying 'no' to invitations without guilt. Do activities that you find enjoyable and relaxing. You can also try proven stress management techniques such as yoga, meditation, and deep breathing exercises.

Develop good sleeping habits

With the right quality and amount of sleep, you can improve your fibro symptoms significantly. Here are some tips to enhance your sleep naturally:

- Set the right mood in your bedroom. Keep it cool, dark, and quiet.

- Keep regular sleeping habits. As much as possible, hit the sack at the same time every night and wake up at the same time every morning, even on weekends or during holidays and vacations.

- Avoid napping in the day as this can interfere with your nighttime sleep. If you really can't help it, minimize your naptime to 1 hour at the most.

- Avoid alcohol and caffeinated drinks in the late afternoon until bedtime.

- Avoid spicy meals or too much intake of liquids before bed. Frequent visits to the bathroom and heartburn can lead to poor sleep quality.

- Don't do anything in your bed but sleep. Reading a thriller, watching late-night shows, or using a laptop in your bed can be stimulating and make it difficult for you to sleep.

- Avoid exercising or doing any physical activity within three hours of sleep time, as it can stimulate you and keep you awake.

- Unwind before bedtime. Do soothing activities like taking a relaxing warm bath or listening to soft, comforting music. A warm bath can also help soothe your aching muscles.

Have a well-balanced diet

Eating the right foods and avoiding toxic ones is one of the best ways to control your symptoms. Inflammatory and acid-forming foods and drinks such as coffee, alcohol, soda, processed food, and fast food can make your body more prone to fatigue and illnesses. Studies also show that an acidic diet interferes with the body's ability to absorb essential nutrients and minerals.

Drink plenty of water

Any form of dehydration can cause headaches, irritability, and disturbed sleep. As there is not enough water to cleanse your system, toxins will accumulate and cause pain in many places, particularly in the muscles and joints.

Start each day with a glass of clean water, preferably on an empty stomach. A standard guideline for water intake is eight 8-ounce glasses per day, but aim to drink more. Aside from rehydrating you, water will detoxify your body and help your muscles recover from fibro flare-ups. It will also increase your energy and improve mental clarity.

Get regular exercise

At first, exercise can increase pain in someone with fibromyalgia. But when you start doing it gradually until it becomes a regular routine, it can decrease your symptoms, reduce stress, help you sleep better, and give you more control over your condition. Start with low-intensity aerobics like walking, biking, swimming, or water aerobics. You can also consult your doctor or a physical therapist to develop a personalized home exercise program. Relaxation techniques, good posture, and stretching are also helpful.

Apply heat or cold for instant relief

Applying heat or cold can ease pain before and/or after a workout. If you feel pain, stiffness, or spasms in your muscles, take a warm bath or use heat lamps, heating pads, or warm wash cloths. Use any of these for 20 minutes, stop for 20 minutes, and then try again.

Overdoing a workout can make you feel sore. A cold compress can provide quick relief by easing swelling and pain. Wrap a cold pack or a small block of ice in a towel so that it isn't in direct contact with your skin. Apply it on the affected area and leave on for about 20 minutes, stop for 20 minutes as well, and then apply again until you feel better.

Don't overthink it

Thinking about your pain too much creates stress and is counterproductive. It may even make you feel more pain than there really is. Being too anxious about your condition increases your cortisol and adrenaline levels, making you more sensitive to feelings of pain. To avoid this, focus on other things like a favorite hobby, a physical activity you enjoy, or anything that can keep your mind from unnecessary thoughts and sensations.

Seek support

Living with chronic pain can be debilitating and extremely difficult. The stigma associated with fibromyalgia and other chronic disorders can make it even harder to cope. But don't be discouraged. If you have fibromyalgia, don't hesitate to seek support. You can find many support groups online and even within your own community. This way, you can get to meet other people who understand you and are going through the same condition. You can encourage and help each other by providing some tips and coping strategies.

You can also go to counselling sessions. A good counselor can talk you into believing in your abilities and boosting your confidence. He or she can also help you better understand your illness, and teach you strategies on how to deal with stressful situations and manage your pain and your condition in general.

Chapter 5: Getting the Right Diet

No drug on the market can beat a healthy, well-balanced diet. Since symptoms of fibromyalgia can be triggered by the food you eat, it is important to be conscious of everything that passes your lips. With a few simple tweaks to your diet, you can lessen the incidence of your symptoms and move more freely and smoothly.

Diet Plans You Can Try

While there is no specific diet designed for fibromyalgia, some diet plans can be helpful as they include a variety of foods that can combat pain and eliminate certain triggers.

First is the anti-inflammatory diet, which is commonly recommended for people with chronic and autoimmune diseases like rheumatoid arthritis, multiple sclerosis, psoriasis, IBS, lupus, and fibromyalgia. This diet focuses on foods that fight inflammation, which is one of the major triggers of fibro symptoms. These include antioxidant-rich foods, essential fatty acids, and mineral-rich foods. On the other hand, it excludes foods that contribute to a leaky gut such as those that are high in trans fat, saturated fat, and refined carbs.

The Mediterranean and DASH Diet (dietary approach to fight hypertension) have also been reported to help people with fibromyalgia. These diets may be helpful in lowering cholesterol and blood pressure, and easing painful symptoms. Many of their components also reduce the amount of inflammation in the body. These two diets have slight differences but both include an abundance of fruits and vegetables, whole grains, legumes, lean proteins, nuts, seeds, and non-fat or low-fat dairy foods.

Foods to Eat

Be optimally healthy and practically pain-free by consuming foods rich in the following:

Omega-3 Fatty Acids

Omega-3 fatty acids have been shown to reduce inflammation, boost immunity, help prevent cardiovascular diseases, and decrease levels of oxidative stress. Oxidative stress occurs when the body is invaded by too many free-radicals, which damage the cells and lead to the development of a number of serious diseases. For people with fibromyalgia and other chronic disorders, omega-3 is particularly helpful in easing painful, tender joints and morning stiffness.

The best sources of omega-3 fatty acids include chia seeds, flaxseeds, walnuts, wild-caught seafood and fatty fish like sardines, salmon, mackerel, tuna, herring, anchovies, and trout. It can also be taken in supplement form. However, try to avoid omega-3 capsules because of their gelatin content. Gelatin contains aspartate and glycine, which are amino acids that activate a certain glutamate receptor in the nerve cells, which can trigger the symptoms of fibromyalgia.

Vitamin D

Studies show that a deficiency in vitamin D can cause pain in the bones and muscles. For people with fibromyalgia who also have this deficiency, vitamin supplementation can aid in easing pain. In a 2008 study, pain patients with poor Vitamin D levels required almost twice the amount of painkillers as compared to those with sufficient levels.

Natural sources of vitamin D include cold-water fish like tuna, swordfish, and sockeye salmon, as well as eggs, milk, and orange juice. It can also be taken in the form of cod liver oil or as a supplement. Spending time in the morning sun also boosts your vitamin D levels, just be sure to wear necessary protection from the harmful rays to reduce your risk of eye disease and skin cancers.

Magnesium

Magnesium helps prevent the excitotoxicity caused by glutamate. Excitotoxicity is a phenomenon in which the levels of neurotransmitters in the neurons initiate cell death. A 2013 study showed that magnesium citrate supplementation was more effective when taken in conjunction with amitriptyline, a try-cyclic antidepressant.

Dark, leafy greens such as spinach, kale, and Swiss chard are excellent sources of magnesium. Legumes (beans and lentils), seeds (e.g. pumpkin seeds), nuts (e.g. almonds), dark chocolate, bananas, avocados, yogurt, and fatty fish are also rich in this nutrient. Have at least three servings of these foods per day to up your magnesium to a healthy level.

Antioxidants

Experts speculate that fibromyalgia symptoms may be caused by oxidative stress, which can worsen if there aren't enough antioxidants in the body. Most fruits and vegetables are rich in important antioxidants including vitamins A, C, and E. These include berries, carrots, beets, kale, spinach, sweet peppers, and others that add various colors to your diet.

Look for food items with vivid red, green, yellow, orange, and purple hues to boost your intake of antioxidants. Whether or not you have fibromyalgia, having adequate antioxidant levels is vital for good health and a long life.

Foods to Avoid

Beware of the following food items. They are known to aggravate fibro symptoms and are best avoided as much as possible.

Artificial Sweeteners

Artificial sweeteners such as aspartame, saccharin, sucralose, and acesulfame-K adversely trigger the neuron receptors, resulting in an increased sensitivity to pain. These food additives are considered *excitotoxins,* which are a class of chemicals that alters brain chemistry and contributes to oxidative stress. Too much of these additives can lead to excitotoxicity, which then can lead to serious neurodegenerative diseases like lupus, Alzheimer's disease, Parkinson's disease, Lou Gehrig's, dementia, and multiple sclerosis.

Aspartame, in particular, has been marketed for years as a "healthy" alternative to sugar, aiding in weight management and weight loss. It can be found in a range of foods and drinks, including yogurts, chewing gums, and diet sodas. In addition to aggravating the pain of fibromyalgia, aspartame contains compounds that have been linked to memory loss, seizures, thyroid conditions, and cancer.

High intake of these sweeteners and additives also increases the risk of diabetes, weight gain, and many other inflammatory diseases. Whereas reducing or eliminating them from your diet has been shown to reduce fibromyalgia symptoms and risk of other health issues.

Refined Carbs (Simple Carbs)

Refined carbs, often found in cookies, pastries, white rice, and white flour, are carbs that are digested quickly in the body. They serve as fast source of energy but cause a sudden and short spike in blood sugar levels. As soon as blood sugar levels drop, you will feel hungry again. Also, this temporary energy boost is often followed by a sudden crash in energy levels. These fluctuations can make pain and fatigue of fibromyalgia worse, and often lead to overeating.

When fibromyalgia leaves you fatigued, it can be tempting to grab some quick sweet treats, but remember that doing so can cause you even more pain. As much as possible, choose whole wheat sources of carbohydrates and natural sources of sugar such as fresh fruits.

Get your dose of complex carbs from whole grains such as whole-wheat berries, wild or brown rice, amaranth, quinoa, and buckwheat oats, or have a plain potato or sweet potato in place of pasta or bread. Whole wheat foods take longer to digest and offer more benefits for the body, whereas refined carbs only increase inflammation.

In addition, too much sugar causes swelling of the nerves as they tend to draw in water. It also reduces flexibility of the outer layer of nerve cells, causing them to rupture and tear. This process ultimately leads to nerve damage which often results in pain, tingling, and numbness in the extremities.

Monosodium Glutamate (MSG)

MSG is a substance used to enhance flavors and preserve foods. It also acts as an excitotoxin molecule that activates neurons in such a way that they increase pain sensitivity. MSG is also loaded with salt, causing aggravation of pain and swelling in many fibromyalgia patients. To minimize the effects of MSG on your condition, avoid prepackaged foods and fast foods as much as possible. Instead, focus on natural whole foods such as brown rice, fatty fish, and lentils.

MSG is commonly present in Chinese foods, frozen dinners, canned soups, mushrooms, tomatoes, potatoes, parmesan cheeses, and many more. Always check the food label for Monosodium Glutamate or MSG. It may also go by other names or be contained in other ingredients but isn't listed separately. Also check these ingredients on labels:

- Glutamate (E 620)

- Glutamic Acid (E 620) 2

- Yeast Extract

- Caseinate

- Gelatin

- Anything hydrolyzed

Also, look out for meat products that include "natural flavor added" on the label. Those natural flavors are sourced from meats, seafood, and plants, and may be high in naturally-occurring MSG.

When eating out, it can be helpful to take note of the restaurants that exclude MSG from their food preparation.

Processed Foods

Processed foods usually have more additives and preservatives, and less nutrients and fiber than unprocessed foods. They also contain unhealthy fats and excessive amounts of sugar. These products include cured, smoked, or canned meats such as sausages, bacon, hotdogs, deli meat, ham, beef jerky and corned beef. Artificial flavorings and preservatives in these foods not only increase inflammation in the body but may also trigger food sensitivities in some people. Always aim for whole real foods like fresh organic vegetables, cage-free eggs, wild-caught fish, and the like.

Unhealthy Fats

Unhealthy fats are present in practically every processed and fried food, as well as in crackers, cookies, doughnuts, and food products that use unhealthy oils during preparation. Certain cheeses and pizzas also contain unhealthy fats and should be avoided. While these foods are convenient and tasty, they are known to worsen symptoms of fibromyalgia.

Unhealthy oils include vegetable oils like safflower, peanut, and corn oils. They trigger inflammation, especially when used to cook or fry food. That's why people with fibromyalgia are advised to remove all sorts of fried foods from their diet. If you cannot entirely get rid of them, use healthier oils, like olive oil, when frying.

Gluten

Whole wheat foods are a healthy alternative to high-carb pastas and white flour breads. However, for people with celiac disease or gluten sensitivity, these foods are best avoided. Gluten is found in wheat, rye, and barley products. Some candies, marinades, and sauces may also contain gluten. Many companies nowadays offer gluten-free food options, so following a gluten-free diet shouldn't be that challenging.

Earlier, whole-wheat foods were recommended as a healthier option over refined carbs, but since celiac disease sometimes overlaps with fibromyalgia, there are some exceptions to the rule. If you suspect you have both conditions, consult your doctor to verify diagnosis and to help you make necessary changes in your diet.

Dairy

Not only can celiac disease overlap with fibromyalgia, but lactose intolerance as well. If you experience symptoms such as gas, bloating, stomach pain, and cramps after eating or drinking dairy products, try eliminating dairy from your diet for a few weeks and see if there's any improvement in your symptoms.

While milk-based products are the primary source of calcium for most people, you can still get this nutrient from calcium-rich alternatives such as soy milk, nuts, broccoli, tuna, and salmon. If you can't completely eliminate dairy, try going only for raw, organic dairy products and avoid pasteurized dairy foods. Some fibromyalgia sufferers find this more tolerable.

It has been shown that a "leaky gut" is the root cause of many chronic conditions and digestive issues. Dairy is one of the major culprits of these problems. Cutting dairy out of your diet can also help with irritable bowel syndrome (IBS) and other digestive disorders.

Nightshades

Nightshades are fruits and vegetables that contain a poisonous compound called *solanine*. This compound naturally occurs in any part of a plant, including the fruit, tubers, and leaves. It is produced by certain plants and has pesticidal and fungicidal properties.

The nightshade family includes tomatoes, white potatoes, eggplant, goji berries, and peppers (chili peppers, bell peppers, cayenne, paprika, pimentos, tomatillos, tamales, etc.). Common symptoms of solanine toxicity include headache, nausea, vomiting, diarrhea, and abdominal pain.

Research shows that 74-90% of people with inflammatory conditions such as fibromyalgia and arthritis experienced increased pain and inflammation after eating fruits and vegetables that belong to the nightshade family. While it is advised to get rid of nightshades altogether, you may try experimenting with these foods to check how your body reacts. But remember to always take everything in moderation.

Red Meat

Red meats are typically high in saturated fats, which can lead to an increased sensitivity to pain, and poor blood circulation. These fats are also risk factors of fatigue. Always opt for white meats like chicken and fish, most especially fatty fish which are rich in omega-3 fatty acids.

Caffeine

Fibromyalgia can cause sleeplessness at night and sleepiness during the day. When you feel fatigued and exhausted, having a cup of coffee or other caffeinated beverages like soda, tea, and energy drinks can be the easiest, most accessible way to get through the day. You might also be tempted to have big bites of your favorite chocolate. However, this can lead to an endless cycle of sleep problems: taking caffeinated drinks to stay awake in the day will keep you from sleeping well at night.

In addition, caffeine increases blood pressure and heart rate, placing even more strain on the muscles. If you cannot get by without coffee or chocolates, keep your intake to minimal amounts, and consume them during the earlier part of the day so they don't interfere with your sleep at night. If possible, always go for healthier alternatives such as an antioxidant-rich, decaffeinated green tea.

It is also important to note that caffeine is sometimes hidden in certain products, such as OTC pain medications, diet pills, and processed foods. Always check the label or list of ingredients when buying.

Alcohol

If your pain and fatigue seem to get worse after consuming alcoholic beverages, then it is best to steer clear of them. Alcohol causes dehydration, which makes the pain in the muscles feel much worse. Alcohol and certain fibromyalgia medications, including antidepressants, anticonvulsants, and drugs containing acetaminophen, can also have harmful interactions.

However, while it worsens pain and fatigue in some people, a research found that moderate alcohol intake can ease symptoms in others. Seek your doctor's advice about the effects of alcohol consumption on your specific situation, even when it doesn't appear to cause flare-ups.

Since fibromyalgia patients react differently to certain foods, it can be a good idea to keep a food diary in which you record what you eat and how you feel after eating it. Does it make your symptoms worse? Does it make you feel better? Or just neutral? Share this food diary with your doctor so you can work together in creating the perfect diet for you.

Chapter 6: 15 Fibro-Friendly Recipes

1. Avocado Egg Toast

Number of Servings: 1

Ingredients:

- Olive oil, for greasing

- 1 clove garlic, grated

- 1 medium egg

- 1 slice whole-grain bread, toasted

- ½ small avocado, smashed

- Red pepper flakes

- Salt and pepper

Directions:

1. Coat a small nonstick skillet with olive oil. Sauté garlic and cook the egg to desired doneness.

2. Spread the smashed avocado over the toasted bread. Add the fried egg on top and sprinkle with salt, pepper, and red pepper flakes. Serve warm.

2. Shiitake Omelet

Number of Servings: 1

Ingredients:

- 2 ½ tsp. coconut oil
- 1 red onion, finely sliced
- 2 handfuls of shiitake mushrooms, sliced
- 2 eggs, whisked
- A pinch of nutmeg
- Salt and pepper, to taste
- Crispy bacon strip
- Cayenne pepper

Directions:

1. Heat oil in a small nonstick skillet. Sauté onions then add the mushrooms. Sprinkle with some salt and nutmeg to taste. Cook over medium heat until the mushrooms are soft.

2. Transfer cooked mushrooms to a bowl. In the same skillet, pour the eggs and cook for 1-2 minutes or until set. Add the mushrooms on one side of the eggs and fold the other half over.

3. Transfer omelet to a serving plate and top with crispy bacon. Sprinkle with cayenne pepper before serving.

3. Hot Quinoa Cereal

Number of Servings: 1

Ingredients:

- 1 cup almond milk, unsweetened
- ¼ cup pomegranate seeds
- 1/3 cup quinoa flakes
- A pinch of sea salt
- Maple syrup, for drizzling
- *Optional toppings*: granola, toasted almonds, toasted walnuts, fresh blueberries, mulberries, goji berries, etc.

Directions:

1. Pour almond milk into a small saucepan over medium-high heat. Bring to a boil.
2. Once boiling, stir in the pomegranate seeds, quinoa flakes, and salt. Turn off heat and stir gently. Let it rest for about 3 minutes, and then stir again to make the cereal thicker.
3. Scoop into a serving bowl and add maple syrup. Serve with your choice of toppings.

4. Chili, Coconut and Pumpkin Soup

Number of Servings: 4

Ingredients:

- 1 tbsp. vegetable oil
- 2.6 lbs. pumpkin, peeled and cut into 2-inch chunks
- 1 carrot, peeled and cut into 2-inch chunks
- 4 cups vegetable stock
- 1 tsp. powdered chili
- 1 red long chili, seeded and chopped
- 1 (165 ml) can coconut cream
- 2 slices day-old white sourdough
- 1 clove garlic, cut in half
- 1 tbsp. butter

Directions:

1. Heat oil in a large stockpot over medium-high heat. Toss in carrots and pumpkin and cook, stirring frequently, until lightly browned, about 3 minutes.

2. Stir in vegetable stock, chili, and powdered chili. Simmer for about 20 minutes, until the vegetables are softened. Turn off heat.

3. Blend the soup mixture with a stick blender. Pour in coconut cream and return to heat. Bring to a boil. Once it has boiled, remove from heat.

4. To make the croutons, rub the garlic on both sides of the sourdough. Be generous so as to give it as much flavor as possible. Slice the bread into 2cm cubes. Heat butter in a nonstick skillet until bubbly. Add the bread cubes and cook, stirring continuously, until crispy and lightly browned on all sides.

5. Ladle soup into separate bowls. Drizzle with more coconut cream and top with a handful of garlic croutons. Serve immediately with extra croutons on the side.

5. Fibro-Healing Soup

Number of Servings: 1

Ingredients:

- 2 tbsp. powdered turmeric

- 2 tbsp. powdered ginger

- 1 tbsp. coconut oil

- 4 cups sodium-free vegetable broth

- 2 stalks scallions, sliced

Directions:

1. Add coconut oil and ginger to a nonstick pan set over medium heat. Whisk until well combined.

2. Pour in the vegetable oil and put to a boil.

3. Reduce heat. Stir in the powdered turmeric and scallions.

4. Ladle into a bowl and serve.

6. Baked Salmon with Herbs

Number of Servings: 4

Ingredients:

- ¼ cup + 2 tbsp. olive oil
- 1.25 lbs. salmon fillet
- Sea salt and ground black pepper
- ¼ cup roughly chopped shallots
- ¼ cup fresh parsley leaves
- ¼ cup fresh dill fronds
- Zest of 1 fresh lemon

Directions:

1. Preheat oven to 250° F.

2. Pour ¼ cup of olive oil into a baking pan then place the salmon fillet, skin-side down, in the oil. Sprinkle with generous amount of salt and ground pepper.

3. In a food processor, add shallots, parsley, dill, and lemon zest and blend until finely chopped. Add in 2 tbsp. of olive oil and pulse until combined. Pat the paste over the fillet.

4. Place the salmon in the preheated oven and bake for 22-28 minutes or until the fish is easily flaked (cooking time may vary depending on the fillet's thickness).

5. Carefully remove the salmon from the pan and onto a cutting board. Cut it into 4 equal parts using a sharp knife.

6. Serve with fresh bread or rice and green salad.

7. Spiced Chicken and Noodles

Number of Servings: 4

Ingredients:

- ¼ tsp. Sichuan peppercorns, finely crushed
- ½ tsp. coarse sea salt
- 2 pods star anise
- ½ cinnamon stick
- ½ tsp. black peppercorns
- 1 4-inch piece fresh ginger, peeled
- 1 3-inch strip orange zest
- 6 ½ cups chicken stock
- Kosher salt
- Freshly ground black pepper
- 4 (6oz each) boneless, skinless chicken breast halves
- 6 shiitake mushrooms, stemmed and thinly sliced
- 3 oz. mung bean noodles
- 2 scallions (green part only), thinly sliced

Directions:

1. Season Sichuan peppercorns with salt. Set aside.
2. Take one inch of the peeled ginger and cut it into thin matchsticks. Cut the remaining 3 inches into fine slices.

3. In a large stockpot, add together chicken stock, star anise, cinnamon stick, black peppercorns, ginger slices, and orange zest. Cover and simmer over medium-low heat for about 20 minutes, or until flavorful and fragrant.

4. Pour the broth through a sieve and into a large pot. Sprinkle with salt and pepper to taste. Return to heat and stir in the mushrooms. Cook on low heat for about 5 minutes or until the mushrooms are tender. Keep the broth covered and hot.

5. Fill a large stockpot with water and simmer the chicken breasts over low heat for about 18 minutes, until the meat is white throughout. Transfer the meat to a cutting board and let sit for 5 minutes. Cut the chicken cross-wise, about 1/2-inch thick. Set aside.

6. Add hot water to a medium bowl and soak the mung bean noodles for 5 minutes or until pliable. Drain and add the noodles to the broth with the mushrooms. Heat through for about a minute.

7. Ladle the soup into separate bowls and top with chicken breasts, ginger matchsticks, and scallions. Sprinkle with the salted Sichuan peppercorns and serve.

8. Baked Tilapia with Pecans

Number of Servings: 4

Ingredients:

- 1/3 cup raw pecans, chopped

- 1/3 cup whole-wheat panko breadcrumbs

- ½ tsp. brown sugar

- 2 tsp. fresh rosemary, chopped

- 1 pinch of cayenne pepper

- 1/8 tsp. salt

- 1 ½ tsp. olive oil

- 1 egg white

- 4 fillets (4oz each) tilapia

Directions:

1. Preheat oven to 350° F.

2. Add pecans, breadcrumbs, brown sugar, rosemary, cayenne pepper, and salt to a small baking dish. Stir together to combine, and then add olive oil. Toss to evenly coat the mixture with oil. Bake for 7-8 minutes or until lightly browned.

3. Add egg white to a shallow dish and whisk vigorously. Dip the tilapia fillets, one at a time, into the egg white then roll over the pecan mixture to lightly coat each side. Lay out the coated fillets in the baking dish.

4. Pour the remaining pecan mix over the fillets and gently press. Bake for about 10 minutes or until cooked through.

5. Remove from the oven and serve hot.

9. Black Bean Burgers

Number of Servings: 6

Ingredients:

- 2 (400g) cans black beans, drained

- 2 tbsp. salted peanuts

- 2 handfuls rolled oats

- Olive oil

- 1 red chili, seeded and finely chopped

- 1 red onion, peeled and coarsely chopped

- 1 tsp. ground cumin

- ½ tsp. ground coriander

- ½ bunch fresh coriander

- Zest of 1 lime, finely grated, plus extra lime for serving

- 1 tsp. sweet smoked paprika

- Plain flour

- 6 bread rolls

- Fresh tomato salsa

- 1 ripe avocado, sliced

- Baby rocket

Directions:

1. Add nuts and oats to a food processor and pulse until coarsely chopped.

2. Add 1½ cans of black beans, chili, onion, ground cumin, ground coriander, coriander leaves, grated lime zest, and a drizzle of olive oil. Pulse again to combine ingredients.

3. Add in the remaining black beans. Pulse only once or twice, so that they stay chunky. Pour mixture into a bowl.

4. Divide the mixture into 6 and form each one into a ball. Place the balls on a clean work surface dusted with smoked paprika and plain flour.

5. Flatten the balls to make burgers, and then lay out the burgers on a tray. Refrigerate for at least 1 hour.

6. Split the bread rolls in half then place them, cut-side down, on a griller. Grill until lightly browned. Set aside.

7. Scatter the baby rocket on 6 of the roll halves. Add the burgers and top with tomato salsa, avocado slices, and rocket. Sandwich with another roll half.

8. Serve with fresh lime cheek for squeezing.

10. Kale Caesar Salad in Chicken Wrap

Number of Servings: 2

Ingredients:

- ½ coddled egg (cooked for 1 minute)
- ½ tsp. Dijon mustard
- 1 tsp. agave syrup
- 1 clove garlic, minced
- 1/8 cup olive oil
- 1/8 cup freshly squeezed lemon juice
- Kosher salt and ground black pepper
- 8 oz. grilled chicken, finely sliced
- 1 cup cherry tomatoes, quartered
- 6 cups curly kale, sliced into bitesize pieces
- ¾ cup parmesan cheese, finely shredded
- 2 lavash flatbreads

Directions:

1. In a medium mixing bowl, combine coddled egg, mustard, agave, garlic, olive oil and lemon juice. Whisk well to make a dressing. Sprinkle with salt and pepper to taste.

2. Stir in chicken, cherry tomatoes, and kale, and toss to coat evenly with the dressing. Add ¼ cup of shredded parmesan.

3. Lay out the 2 flatbreads. Spread even amounts of the salad over each wrap and sprinkle with the remaining parmesan cheese.

4. Roll up the chicken wraps and cut in half. Serve immediately.

11. Chickpea Salad

Number of Servings: 6

Ingredients:

- 1 large cucumber, seeded and cubed
- 2 cups grape tomatoes, halved
- 1 (15 oz.) can chickpeas, drained and rinsed
- 1 orange bell pepper, seeded and chopped
- 1 red bell pepper, seeded and chopped
- 5 scallions (both green and white parts), diced
- ¼ cup minced mint leaves
- ¼ cup minced flatleaf parsley
- ½ cup + ¼ cup crumbled feta cheese

For the vinaigrette

- Juice and zest of 3 fresh lemons
- 1 clove garlic, grated
- 2 tsp. basil paste
- ½ cup olive oil
- 1 tsp. kosher salt
- ½ tsp. freshly ground black pepper
- Toasted pita chips

Directions:

1. Mix together cucumber, grape tomatoes, chickpeas, bell peppers, scallions, mint, parsley, and ½ cup crumbled feta in a large mixing bowl.

2. In a separate small bowl, add lemon juice and zest, garlic, and basil paste, and whisk together to combine.

3. Slowly pour in olive oil, whisking, until everything is emulsified. Season with salt and black pepper and whisk well to make the vinaigrette. Pour this over the veggies and toss gently to combine.

4. Top with the remaining feta cheese and serve with pita chips.

12. Granola and Seeds Mix

Number of Servings: 4

Ingredients:

- ¼ cup extra-virgin olive oil
- ¼ cup unsalted butter
- 2 tbsp. honey
- 2 cups almonds
- 4 cups oats
- ½ cup sunflower seeds
- ¾ cup pumpkin seeds
- 1 tsp. cinnamon

Directions:

1. Preheat oven to 350° F.

2. Cook oil, butter, and honey in a small nonstick saucepan set over low heat.

3. In a large mixing bowl, stir together all the remaining ingredients. Pour the oil and butter mixture over the seeds and granola mixture. Stir until well combined.

4. Place the mixture on a baking sheet, spread evenly. Bake until the granola is browned, for about 1 hour. Turn and stir the mixture gently every 20 minutes while baking.

5. Remove from oven and transfer to individual serving bowls. Serve warm.

13. Kale Chips

Ingredients:

- 1 head kale, stemmed
- ½ tsp. turmeric
- 1 tbsp. olive oil

Directions:

1. Preheat oven to 275° F.

2. Tear the kale leaves into chip-size pieces. Wash thoroughly and let dry completely. (Make sure the leaves are totally dry before baking; wet leaves will make soggy chips.)

3. On a parchment paper-lined cookie sheet, spread kale in a single layer. Be sure they don't pile up over each other. Sprinkle with turmeric and drizzle with olive oil.

4. Bake in the oven for 10 minutes. Rotate the cookie sheet then bake again for 10-15 minutes, until the edges of the leaves are browned.

5. Take out of the oven and let cool for 3 minutes before serving. Enjoy!

14. Pain-Relieving Cocoa Smoothie

Number of Servings: 1

Ingredients:

- 1 cup almond milk
- 1 tbsp. cocoa powder, unsweetened
- 2 tbsp. oatmeal
- 1 tbsp. powdered barley grass
- ½ cup spinach
- Whipped cream
- Cocoa beans

Directions:

1. Add all the ingredients to a blender and process until smooth.
2. Transfer to a tall glass and add whipped cream. Top with cocoa beans and serve.

15. Homemade Ginger Ale

Ingredients:

- 2 cups purified water
- 1 cup ginger, peeled and finely chopped
- Sparkling water

- Juice of 1 lemon

- Raw honey

Directions:

1. Add water to a small pot and put to a boil. Add ginger, and then reduce heat to medium-low. Let simmer for about 5 minutes.

2. Remove from heat and strain. To serve, combine 1 part ginger mixture and 3 parts sparkling water. Add lemon juice and raw honey to sweeten taste. Serve on the rocks.

Chapter 7: Best Exercises for Fibromyalgia

When your body aches all over, the last thing you would want to do is to move a lot and exercise. But according to research, performing physical activities on a regular basis is instrumental to easing many fibromyalgia symptoms. You don't need to run marathons or lift heavy weights to reap the benefits of exercise. You can start with a gentle approach to slowly increase your stamina and restore your flexibility.

Choose an exercise you enjoy so you can keep yourself motivated to go out and get moving. Here are the best exercises you can do to reduce pain flare-ups and have a more enjoyable day-to-day life.

Walking

One of the easiest yet most effective ways to get into exercise is to go for a walk. It doesn't need to be a long or vigorous one. You can start with 10-20 minutes per day—even 5 minutes if that's too much for you—at your own pace, then gradually work up to 30 minutes per day. You can also run to increase the pace if you feel up to it.

Walk your dog if that motivates you, or take your whole family for a nice walk around the neighborhood. If possible, incorporate some inclined hills to further activate your muscles while walking. To help you stay on track, you may also join a workout or walking group in your community.

Walking is an excellent form of light aerobics as it provides a number of healing benefits: boosts energy, reduces pain and stiffness, helps restore stamina, brings nutrition and oxygen to the muscles, and strengthens the bones. Instead of doing long stretches, people with fibromyalgia can break them up into shorter chunks so as to relax the muscles every now and then.

Either way, the health benefits are the same. Aim to do some light aerobics 3 to 4 times per week.

Stretching

Daily stretching can help the joints move with more ease—often referred to as the range of motion. Stretching helps release pain and stiffness by elongating your muscles. It increases your flexibility, loosens tight muscles, and helps you get better sleep at night. When stretching, focus on the muscle groups that are most affected by fibromyalgia: shoulders, lower and mid back, hips, thighs, and calves. Hold the stretches for 10-30 seconds but stop it if hurts.

Have a good stretch at least once per day. This will help you with your day-to-day activities, such as cooking, cleaning, driving, gardening, and shopping. Stretching during a workout can also help you tolerate your training better.

Biking

Biking is another form of light aerobics that provides plenty of health benefits. The back-and-forth, reciprocal motion helps with relaxation and eases tension in the muscles. A bike ride moves your lower body without straining it. Your joints and muscles will start to warm up and move more smoothly the longer you ride.

If you're a beginner, you can start biking on paved roads for shorter periods, then gradually move up to longer excursions on more challenging roads, like up-hills. If you live close to your office, consider riding your bike to work.

Swimming

Swimming is another excellent low-impact aerobics that is ideal for fibromyalgia patients. Water offers both support and resistance for the body, and a meditative experience for the mind. It improves range of motion, while being gentle on the joints and muscles. If you like the idea of swimming, consider water aerobics in a heated pool. Cold water stiffens the muscles, but warm water relaxes the muscles and relieves it of aches.

Strength Training

Pained muscles may flinch at first with strength training, but this type of exercise is important for your overall physical fitness. Move slowly, if necessary, or use lighter weights to begin with. You can start using 1-3-pound dumbbells and lift slowly but precisely in order to strengthen muscles and improve tone. If you don't have weights, grab a couple of bottled or canned goods to get started.

Stronger muscles are less prone to fatigue. Studies also suggest that strength training can help with depression as effectively as some medications. Make it a goal to train each major area—abs, arms, back, shoulders, chest, and legs—2 or 3 times per week.

You can start by doing 8 repetitions with a weight you can comfortably lift, then work up to 10-12 repetitions. Once you can work with a heavier weight (increase the weight slightly at certain intervals), start again at 8 repetitions then work up to 12, and so on.

Group Exercises

Joining group exercises can help you stay motivated. You can join an aerobics, low-intensity yoga, or tai chi class and work people who are also eager to improve their health. Some recreation and fitness centers also offer group exercise classes dedicated to people with chronic pain and low mobility. These classes provide a comfortable and safe environment for anyone who's just getting started with their workouts, or is dealing with taxing symptoms.

Yoga

Yoga offers mind-body awareness, gentle stretching, and a low-impact approach to strengthening all the muscle groups in the body. A study shows that yoga can be helpful for alleviating many fibromyalgia symptoms, including muscle pain and stiffness, depression, perceived disability, and restricted movement.

According to a research published in the Journal of Pain Research, yoga reduces both psychological and physical symptoms of fibro as it offers meditation, as well as breathing techniques and a gentle combination of various postures. Yoga also helps to properly realign the bones so that the skeleton provides more support to the body.

This practice is easily accessible, as many gyms, community centers, and fitness centers offer yoga classes. You will also find many free yoga videos online, including some that are specifically designed for chronic pain. Aim to incorporate a simple 20-minute yoga session, even in the comfort of your home, into your routine, and you can be well on your way to better physical and mental health.

Daily Activities

Doing your daily activities counts, too! Studies show that everyday activities like mopping the floors, mowing the yard, cleaning windows, gardening, playing with your kids and grandkids, and just about anything that gets you moving counts toward reducing your symptoms and increasing physical fitness. But as always, listen to your body. If you're doing a chore and feel pain, or are playing with your kids but it strains your muscles, stop and take a rest.

Benefits of Exercise for Fibromyalgia

Need more motivation to get going? Read these wonderful benefits you can gain from a simple exercise regimen.

- **Eases pain naturally**

Regular exercise has been shown to combat pain as well as some prescription medicines. Recent studies show that there is no significant difference between the pain relief achieved from non-opioid analgesics, and that achieved from routine exercise. While exercise can take more time to relieve pain, it is free and has no side-effects.

Exercise also has a positive impact on the way the brain processes pain. It's been mentioned before that fibromyalgia may be due to the brain lowering the pain threshold or misinterpreting the pain signals, causing unnecessary aches. Exercise may be able to reverse this and modify the course of the condition.

- **Increases energy**

Less pain means more energy. Exercise increases your heart rate and keeps your blood pumping, giving you that oomph to get up and go. The more you intensify your workouts, the more you will feel energized and less fatigued.

- **Reduces the effects of depression**

People with fibromyalgia generally have low levels of serotonin, which often results in depression. The good news is that exercise increases serotonin levels in the brain, and thereby reduces the effects of depression and makes you feel happier. Serotonin is the feel-good hormone that boosts mood and promotes greater feelings of wellbeing.

Regular exercise also increases the production of endorphins, which are chemicals in the brain that decrease your perception of pain, leaving you feeling more positive and euphoric–a feeling often referred to as the "runner's high." Endorphins also act as sedatives, without the dangers of dependence or addiction.

- **Sharpens memory and thinking**

  Aside from making you feel better, endorphins can also improve your concentration and sharpen mental functions. They make you more alert and efficient at performing any tasks at hand. Exercise can also help prevent age-related degeneration, and stimulate the birth of new brain cells.

- **Lowers cortisol levels**

  Chronic pain can lead to chronic stress, which then can lead to a number of other health issues. Exercise can help by aiding in relaxation and helping to manage cortisol levels.

  High levels of cortisol are associated with increased levels of stress. Performing regular physical activities stimulates the production of both adrenaline and cortisol at the beginning, and drops both at the end. Boost this effect by doing some light to moderate exercise in the morning, when cortisol levels are the highest, and benefit from its calming effects for the most part of the day.

- **Improves sleep**

  People with fibromyalgia often suffer from sleep disorders which can further aggravate pain. You can fight this by getting into a good exercise routine. Any form of physical activity can promote longer restorative and better-quality sleep, which in turn helps to ease pain. Even a short burst of light exercise in the morning or afternoon can help in regulating sleep patterns.

- **Improves the immune system**

  Having a stronger immune system makes you less prone to colds, the flu, and other viruses. Exercising encourages the cells in the immune system to work faster and harder in fighting germs and bacteria that cause various infections and illnesses.

- **Boosts self-esteem**

One of the key psychological benefits of regular exercise is increased self-esteem. Endorphins are partly responsible for this. Moreover, meeting exercise challenges or fitness goals, even just small ones, can boost your sense of self-worth and foster your self-confidence. Getting in good shape will also make you feel better about yourself and your appearance.

- **Improves resilience**

When faced with life difficulties, many people resort to drugs, alcohol, and other negative habits, which, instead of fixing the problem, only worsen the situation. Turning to exercise helps you cope with emotional or mental challenges in a healthy way. It helps you stay away from negative behaviors while reducing your symptoms and improving your general health.

- **Increases social interaction**

Engaging in exercise and other physical activities gives you the opportunity to socialize with other people. Greeting your neighbors as you walk around the block, or exchanging friendly smiles can lift your mood. Joining classes in the gym or community center also gives you the chance to meet new friends and become more sociable.

With these amazing benefits, exercise can be extremely helpful not only for people with fibromyalgia or mood disorders, but also for those who are suffering from other conditions such as arthritis, diabetes, high blood pressure, and other forms of chronic pain. And even if you don't have any of these diseases, being physically active and having a good lifestyle is vital to achieve optimal health and a more positive outlook in life.

Chapter 8: Essential Oils for Instant Comfort

Essential oils are known for their immense therapeutic benefits which can be extremely helpful for people with chronic pain. Using these oils is another easy and convenient way to reduce your symptoms. Some of the best essential oils for fibromyalgia include:

Lavender Oil

Lavender is widely known for its calming and stress-relieving properties. It has a number of medicinal uses, including being a powerful pain relief agent. Lavender oil is antidepressant, anti-inflammatory, antiseptic, antispasmodic, and analgesic. These properties make it an ideal choice for muscle pain, back pain, rheumatism, cramps, arthritis, nausea, headaches, and fibromyalgia. It calms the nerves, helps improve blood circulation, and relieves stress, depression, anxiety, and nervous exhaustion. Lavender oil is also an excellent sleep aid.

Peppermint Oil

Peppermint has a minty fragrance which makes it a popular ingredient for toothpastes and cough syrups. Its oil is an effective analgesic (for inducing sleep), anti-inflammatory (for reducing pains and aches), and antispasmodic (for relieving muscle cramps and spasms). Its fresh scent can also help reduce fatigue and clear fibro fog.

Other benefits include boosting the nervous system, easing pain sensitivity from headaches, improving memory, reducing congestion, and helping with breathing conditions like asthma. It has also been found to be a temporary cure for irritable bowel syndrome.

Eucalyptus Oil

Inflammation and poor blood circulation are the main causes of muscle soreness and aches, and the build-up of toxins and other harmful substances in the body. Eucalyptus is your choice of oil for tackling these issues. This oil helps reduce fibro flare-ups by promoting good blood circulation, fighting inflammation, and helping to flush toxins out of the body. Its analgesic and anti-inflammatory properties can also provide instant relief from body aches, ease fatigue, boost mood, and invigorate the spirit.

Helichrysum Oil

Helichrysum oil is effective for relieving tension and stress, reducing fatigue, and improving blood circulation. It has anti-inflammatory, antioxidant, analgesic, and antidepressant properties. It is a promising oil for decreasing pain by easing inflammation and swelling. Helichrysum can also correct pain disorders and help soothe the nervous system.

Sandalwood Oil

Sandalwood is an aromatic tree whose oil is widely used for its anti-inflammatory and antiseptic effects. It's also known for its ability to sedate and calm the nerves. Sandalwood contains the compound *santalol*, which is shown to have depressant and sedative effects on the body's central nervous system. A 2007 study shows that sandalwood oil, when inhaled, improves sleep and promotes non-rapid eye movement (NREM) sleep.

Rosemary Oil

There is a reason rosemary is known as the "herb of remembrance." The oil extracted from this herb has been shown to enhance memory by stimulating the nerve growth factor, and assisting in the healing process of neurological tissues. Aside from promoting mental alertness and reducing fibro fog, rosemary also has high analgesic properties, making it effective for easing pain in the muscles and joints. You can also use it for nausea, headaches, back pain, rheumatism, and as a sleep aid.

Ginger Oil

More than being an ingredient for cooking, ginger is a potent anti-inflammatory agent. It effectively relieves spasms, reduces nausea, and blocks pain sensations. Its antidepressant and analgesic properties offer relief from joint and muscle pains, arthritis, and inflammation. Aside from these benefits, ginger can also improve blood circulation, aid digestion, and detoxify the body. It has also been reported to stimulate the activity of antioxidants in the body.

Black Pepper Oil

Black pepper oil is one of the best essential oils for muscle pains and aches. It warms the muscles, therefore improving circulation and increasing body heat which is good for the muscles and nerves. More than being an excellent pain reliever, black pepper oil is also used as a stress reliever, an immunity booster, and a digestive aid. People with fibromyalgia, rheumatism, and arthritis will find it to be an outstanding companion. This is a strong oil, so avoid applying it directly to the skin, and use it sparingly.

How to Use Essential Oils

There are several ways to use essential oils, including:

Topical application: Applying diluted essential oil on various trigger points provides significant relief from pain. You can apply the oil yourself, or use it during massage or physical therapy.

Aromatherapy: This involves aerating or diffusing essential oils so that you can inhale their aroma, which will relieve your stress and soothe your nerves. Use an oil diffuser to conveniently ease your pain, anxiety, and insomnia.

Hot bath: Adding essential oils to your bath soothes your muscles and allows the oil to be absorbed into your skin, while inhaling the steam provides the benefits of aromatherapy. The warm water will also improve your circulation, which helps reduce pain.

Before applying essential oil to your skin, make sure to dilute it with a carrier oil. This is to minimize potency and prevent skin irritation. Dilute 3-5 drops of your preferred essential oil in an ounce of any of these carrier oils:

- olive oil
- almond oil
- coconut oil
- grapeseed oil
- avocado oil
- massage oils
- unscented lotions

As many essential oils are toxic, they should not be taken orally. Before using essential oils for fibromyalgia, discuss the risks and benefits with your doctor.

Conclusion

Thanks again for choosing this book!

I hope you enjoyed learning more about Fibromyalgia, and found this book to be helpful.

If you enjoyed this book, please take the time to leave me a review on Amazon. I appreciate your honest feedback, and it really helps me to continue producing high quality books.

Lightning Source UK Ltd.
Milton Keynes UK
UKHW020634150120
357000UK00011B/273/P